BACK PAIN EXERCISE FOR WOMEN OVER 60

The Complete Step by Step Guide to Getting Rid of Lower and Upper Back ache through easy and mild yoga, Pilates and stretching in order to Achieve Good Health

Brett Switzer

1

TABLE OF CONTENT

INTRODUCTION

Margaret was a great woman who lived in a charming village where the dusk sky created a calm painting. Margaret was sixty years old and had persevered through many hardships in life.

However, nothing had affected her as much as the chronic upper and lower back discomfort that had plagued her for years. It was an imperceptible restraint preventing her from living a rich and active life. Margaret, nevertheless, did not give up lightly.

The narrative of Margaret's resiliency and rejuvenation surfaced in a book called "Back Pain Exercise for Women Over 60." This book turned into her lighthouse, providing a route to a better, pain-free life designed especially for women in their 60s with chronic back pain.

When Margaret was diagnosed with osteoarthritis in her early 50s, it was a disheartening diagnosis that set off her fight with back discomfort.

Although Margaret knew she might have surgery, she was determined to look into other options.

She yearned for a remedy that would not only ease her suffering but also revitalize her body and soul, and she discovered the solutions she was looking for in the book's pages.

Margaret was determined to live a pain-free, healthier life, so she followed the professional advice in "Back Pain Exercise for Women Over 60."

She began her morning routines with the mild exercises suggested in the book, emphasizing posture correction, flexibility improvement, and core muscle development. Margaret found comfort in the routine's simplicity every day as the sun caressed her garden. By walking, doing yoga, and stretching, she was able to gradually regain her balance.

Margaret's metamorphosis was nothing short of amazing as the weeks stretched into months. Her back discomfort subsided with time, and she felt more energetic than ever.

The simple yet effective workouts she had followed in the book had completely transformed her body. Margaret became more confident and her posture straightened. Family and friends noticed the change in her physical appearance as well as the brightness of her attitude.

The sparkle in her eyes, though, was the biggest difference. Margaret was not just pain-free but also fully engaged in life. She started taking part in neighborhood activities, picking up old pastimes, and even taking up gardening, a love she had long wanted to pursue again. Her narrative became an inspiration to many, and her laughter filled the community.

Margaret's trip was a tour of self-discovery as much as it was about getting over her back discomfort. She demonstrated that living a full life should never be impeded by one's age.

Her experience proved that happiness, excellent posture, and good health could be regained with hard work and the correct advice from "Back Pain Exercise for Women Over 60."

Margaret had turned a new page in her life, one that she had written with the exercises and resilience ink suggested in the book.

In the end, Margaret's narrative offers hope and encouragement to any woman over 60 who may be struggling with lower back pain, since it is guided by the knowledge found in the book.

They too may enjoy the joys of a pain-free, active, and fulfilling life with the right exercises, perseverance, and steadfast determination just like the narrative found in "Back Pain Exercise for Women Over 60."

Margaret's journey, one chapter at a time, serves as a reminder that it is never too late to recover one's happiness and health.

Chapter 1: Overview of Back Pain

All ages are commonly affected by back discomfort, but women over 60 may find it more difficult to manage. Due to natural degenerative changes in the spine with age, back discomfort is more common in older women.

The good news is that, for those in this age range, regular exercise may be extremely important for both controlling and avoiding back discomfort.

It's important to identify the particular elements that contribute to women over 60's sensitivity to back pain in order to appreciate the importance of back pain exercises.

Age-related conditions such as osteoporosis, decreased muscle mass, and decreased flexibility can make back discomfort worse in older women. Hormonal changes can also weaken bones and make them more prone to fracture, such as a drop in estrogen after menopause.

Proper back pain exercises can help reduce pain and enhance one's quality of life in general.

The main goal of these exercises should be to strengthen the muscles of the back, abdomen, and pelvis, together known as the core.

Walking, swimming, and tai chi are examples of low-impact exercises that can help with balance and posture, two important factors in the prevention of back pain.

Older women can benefit from yoga and pilates as well since they improve core strength and flexibility. Deep breathing exercises and mild stretches can help promote relaxation and the release of back tightness. It is imperative that you begin softly and increase the intensity gradually in order to prevent overexertion.

It is also essential to speak with a medical expert or physical therapist in order to customize an exercise program for back pain to suit the unique demands and limits of each individual.

To guarantee security and efficacy, they may offer tailored advice.

Due to age-related changes, back pain is a major worry for women over 60. However, exercise can be an effective technique for managing and preventing back pain.

Exercise regimens specifically designed to target core strength, flexibility, and general well-being can significantly enhance the quality of life and minimize back pain in older women, enabling them to enjoy their later years.

Risk factors and causes

Back discomfort is a common condition that can have a major impact on one's quality of life, particularly for women who are over 60.

When creating workout regimens to reduce discomfort and stop more problems, it is essential to comprehend the risk variables and causes of back pain in this population.

Age-related degeneration of the spine is a major risk factor for back pain in women over sixty.

The discs between our vertebrae grow less flexible and lose moisture as we age, making us more susceptible to damage.

Furthermore, osteoporosis, a disorder that weakens the bones, can increase the risk of compression fractures and fractures in the spine, both of which can exacerbate back discomfort.

Lack of exercise and sedentary lifestyles are two more prevalent reasons for back pain.

This age group of women may have worked for years at desk occupations or performing low-physical-demanding home tasks. Poor posture and weak core muscles can put additional strain on the back and make discomfort worse.

Obesity, smoking, and a history of illnesses like herniated discs or arthritis are additional risk factors. It's critical to understand that each person's back discomfort may have a different cause.

One useful tactic for controlling and avoiding back pain is exercise. Low-impact exercises that enhance flexibility, strength, and posture for women over 60 include swimming, strolling, and mild yoga.

Exercises that strengthen the core are very beneficial for maintaining spinal stability.

Before beginning any workout program, it is imperative to speak with a healthcare professional or a physical therapist, as they can customize the regimen to each person's wants and circumstances, guaranteeing a secure and efficient method of treating back pain.

The Value of Physical Activity

Engaging in physical exercise is crucial for managing and avoiding back pain, particularly for women who are over 60.

Natural changes that occur to our bodies as we age include a loss of bone density, flexibility, and muscle mass, all of which can aggravate back discomfort.

Regular, individually tailored physical activity can dramatically enhance an older woman's general health and quality of life while lowering her risk of developing back discomfort.

Maintaining the strength of the back and core muscles which are critical for supporting the spine and avoiding strain requires regular exercise.

Combining strength training, flexibility exercises, and low-impact cardiovascular activities can be beneficial for women over 60. By assisting in the growth and maintenance of muscle mass, strength training can reduce strain on the spine.

Tai chi and yoga are examples of flexibility activities that can improve range of motion and lower the risk of injury.

Walking and swimming are examples of low-impact cardiovascular exercises that can help control weight and enhance cardiovascular health, both of which are important for managing back pain.

Additionally, exercise encourages the release of endorphins, which are endogenous analgesics; additionally, exercise can elevate mood and lower stress levels, all of which are known to increase back pain.

Additionally, it can help keep a healthy body weight, which lessens the tension on the back even more.

To sum up, exercise is a crucial tool for women over 60 to control and avoid back discomfort.

Personalized exercise programs may improve physical strength, flexibility, and general well-being when paired with a healthy lifestyle. This can pave the way for an active and pain-free golden age.

Chapter 2: Get Ready for a Safe Workout

A healthy lifestyle must include exercise, particularly for women over 60. But it's crucial for those with back pain to approach exercise cautiously and put safety first.

This is a handbook for women over 60 who want to manage their back pain and be ready for a safe and successful fitness program.

Speak with a Medical Professional: It's important to speak with a medical professional before beginning any workout program.

Ideally, this person will specialize in physical therapy or orthopedics. They are able to evaluate your particular case of back pain and provide customized advice.

20

Gentle Warm-Up: To prepare your muscles and lower your chance of injury, start every workout with a gentle warm-up.

Put your attention on low-impact exercises like light stretching or walking. It's especially crucial for elderly people with back discomfort to warm up.

Core Strengthening: Your back can receive much-needed support from a strong core. Include exercises that strengthen the core, such as leg lifts, planks, and pelvic tilts. Back pain can be reduced and spine stability can be achieved with these exercises.

Low-Impact Cardio: To increase general fitness, take part in low-impact cardiovascular workouts.

Effective cardiovascular exercises that are less taxing on the back include swimming, stationary cycling, and water aerobics.

Stretching regularly might help you become more flexible and lower your chance of spraining your muscles.

Add back-specific workouts to your routine, such as Tai Chi or mild yoga. These exercises encourage pain alleviation and relaxation.

Exercise with mindfulness by paying great attention to your body's cues. Exercise should be modified or stopped right away if it hurts or causes discomfort. Pay attention to what your body tells you, then modify your regimen.

Posture Awareness: Keeping a healthy posture both in everyday life and during exercise is essential for managing back pain. Pay attention to your posture, whether you're working out, sitting, or standing.

Gradual Progression: Do not overextend yourself too quickly.To avoid overexerting yourself and to give your body time to adjust, gradually increase the duration and intensity of your workouts.

Cool down and Stretch: To minimize muscular discomfort and promote healing, spend some time cooling down and stretching after your workout.

Maintain Proper Hydration and Nutrition: In addition to being beneficial for general health, proper diet and hydration can also help avoid injuries and speed up recovery.

Keep in mind that each woman has a different back pain problem, so creating a customized workout program with your healthcare physician and a certified fitness trainer is essential.

Women over 60 can safely and successfully manage their back pain while reaping the many advantages of regular exercise if they take the appropriate approach.

Seeking Advice from a Medical Professional

Many individuals worry about back discomfort, but as women age, it can provide unique challenges.

Even though it's commonly said that exercise could relieve back discomfort, ladies over a certain age should consult a doctor before beginning any fitness program.

 By following this advice, you may be sure that the workouts you've selected are both safe and suitable for your requirements.

Numerous conditions, such as osteoporosis, degenerative disc disease, or even muscle imbalances, can result in back discomfort in older women.

Different methods and exercises may be needed for certain illnesses in order to reduce pain.

Finding the source of your back discomfort and creating a suitable fitness program require speaking with a medical expert, such as a physical therapist or primary care physician.

Medical practitioners can offer tailored advice depending on a patient's objectives, physical restrictions, and current state of health.

They can also assist in tracking development and modifying the workout regimen as needed. They can also offer guidance on how to exercise properly and avoid injury.

Additionally, some older women may already be dealing with medical issues that might affect how they choose to exercise.

For example, to guarantee their safety, those with diabetes or heart issues may need to perform modified activities. Experts in medicine can offer advice on how to modify activities to take these health issues into account.

The best course of action for older ladies experiencing back discomfort is to consult a medical practitioner.

They provide the knowledge and experience required to create a customized workout program that not only reduces back pain but also enhances general health and wellbeing.

In order to achieve these goals, safety and efficacy must come first, and a medical professional's advice is priceless.

Evaluating Your Degree of Fitness

Keeping up physical fitness is essential for general health and wellbeing, and it gets more important as we get older.

As they approach their senior years, women in particular confront distinct difficulties, such as a higher chance of back discomfort.

Back discomfort can be crippling, impairing everyday activities, and restricting range of motion. Regular back-healthy activity, however, can help reduce discomfort and enhance quality of life.

Assessing your level of back pain exercise readiness is a proactive measure to make sure you stay pain-free and active as you age. To begin, take into account the following elements:

Medical Evaluation: Speak with your healthcare professional before starting any fitness regimen. They are able to evaluate your present state of health, detect any underlying issues, and provide recommendations based on your individual requirements.

Range of Motion: Evaluate your range of motion and flexibility. Being stiff is frequently linked to back discomfort. Stretching gently can increase flexibility and lower the chance of strained muscles.

Strength: Assess the strength of your muscles, particularly those in your back and core. By making these muscles stronger, you can lower your chance of developing back discomfort and provide your spine more support.

Posture: Be mindful of your alignment. Back discomfort can be exacerbated by bad posture. To reduce strain on your spine, maintain proper posture when performing regular tasks and exercising.

Exercises for balance and stability are vital because they reduce the risk of falls and the injuries they cause. Make sure your regimen includes workouts that test your stability and balance.

Cardiovascular Fitness: Engage in physical activities such as swimming or brisk walking to maintain your cardiovascular health. Enhancing blood circulation to the spine through a healthy heart might facilitate the healing process.

Monitoring Pain: Be mindful of any soreness or discomfort both during and after physical activity. While some degree of muscular soreness is common, chronic or escalating discomfort has to be treated right once.

Keep in mind that while assessing your level of fitness for managing back pain, consistency is essential.

As you increase the intensity of your workout, don't push yourself too hard too quickly. If necessary, get advice from a certified fitness specialist with experience in back pain exercises.

As you become older, back discomfort doesn't have to keep you from living the life you want.

You may strengthen your back, increase mobility, and live a better quality of life as a woman over 60 by determining your current level of fitness and putting into practice a comprehensive exercise program.

Selecting the Proper Exercise Equipment

Choosing the right workout equipment for back pain alleviation is crucial for women who want to keep their bodies in good shape as they age.

Women over 60 may frequently have back pain, but with the correct tools and exercise routine, back pain may be reduced and general back health can be enhanced.

It is crucial to give low-impact solutions first priority when selecting workout equipment. Elliptical machines, stationary cycles, and treadmills are great options for cardiovascular exercises that don't overly strain the back.

These devices provide smooth, regulated motions that lower the chance of damage while strengthening the muscles that support the spine.

Strength training is yet another essential part of treating back pain. Targeted muscle strengthening is made possible by cable machines, dumbbells, and resistance bands.

Building core strength is especially important for women over 60, since it can dramatically alleviate back discomfort by improving spinal support.

Select training equipment that allows you to target different muscle areas with a range of routines.

Enhancing flexibility and balance are critical for preventing back discomfort, and both may be achieved with yoga and pilates.

You only need a yoga mat and a few props, such blocks and straps, for these exercises.

They can aid in lowering back muscle tension and enhancing spinal mobility.

Finally, think about spending money on a stability ball. It's a flexible piece of equipment that can help with workouts for balance and core strength.

Additionally, sitting on a stability ball might aid with posture, which is crucial for lowering back discomfort.

Before starting any training program, it's essential to speak with a healthcare provider or a competent fitness trainer regardless of the equipment you use, particularly if you already have back problems.

They may provide you individualized advice on the activities and equipment that will best suit your needs.

Choosing the appropriate workout equipment is essential for ladies who want to control their back discomfort.

Enhancing one's quality of life and back health can be achieved by integrating flexibility and balance exercises, strength training, and low-impact choices.

Chapter 3: Mild Mobility and Stretching Exercises

Back discomfort is a typical complaint, especially as we become older. However, for women, back pain can grow more severe with time owing to a variety of reasons such as osteoporosis, muscle mass loss, and the natural aging process.

Mild mobility and stretching exercises are an excellent strategy to manage and relieve back discomfort. These exercises can help increase flexibility, strengthen muscles, and alleviate back pain.

Gentle stretching exercises are an excellent place to start for ladies suffering from back discomfort.

Neck stretches, shoulder rolls, and moderate back twists are all simple routines that can help reduce stress and increase mobility. Regularly performing these exercises can keep muscles from getting excessively tight and causing pain.

Yoga and Pilates are wonderful alternatives for ladies who want to improve their flexibility and core strength.

These exercises emphasize regulated motions and mild stretching, which can be very good for the elderly.

There are several courses and DVDs available that cater to all fitness levels, ensuring that ladies can find a regimen that works for them.

Swimming is another fantastic choice. Water's buoyancy lowers the strain on the spine while offering a full-body exercise.

Water aerobics, in particular, may be an enjoyable way to keep active while also relieving back discomfort.

Tai Chi, sometimes known as "meditation in motion," mixes slow, flowing motions and deep breathing.

It's a great option for increasing balance and flexibility, both of which can help relieve back discomfort and lower the chance of falling.

Incorporating these gentle mobility and stretching exercises into a daily regimen can help women manage their back discomfort significantly.

However, before beginning any new fitness program, it is critical to contact a healthcare practitioner or physical therapist, especially if you have an existing medical problem.

You may increase your mobility, reduce back discomfort, and have a better quality of life by personalizing an exercise plan to your unique needs.

Shoulder and Neck Extension

Aches and pains are normal as we get older, especially in the back and neck.

Women, in particular, have additional obstacles as a result of a variety of variables, such as posture, muscular weakness, and lower bone density.

Shoulder and neck extensions are a helpful workout for relieving these discomforts.

This workout focuses on the upper body, which helps to improve posture and minimize tension in the back and neck.

To avoid and treat back discomfort, women over the age of 60 must maintain proper posture and mobility.

Follow these instructions to conduct Shoulder and Neck Extensions:

Sit or stand tall, your feet shoulder-width apart.

Relax your neck and gently drop your shoulders.

Lift your shoulders slowly upward towards your ears, as if shrugging, and hold for a few seconds.

Relax by lowering your shoulders again.

Repeat this motion for about 10-15 times.

This exercise is advantageous for various reasons:

Posture Correction: Women over the age of 60 may slouch, putting additional strain on the back and neck. Shoulder and neck

40

extensions aid in maintaining a more upright posture.

Neck discomfort Relief: Many elderly persons suffer from neck discomfort as a result of tension and poor posture. This exercise might help you feel better by stretching and strengthening your neck muscles.

Stress Reduction: The soothing motion of the exercise can also aid in the reduction of stress and tension, both of which can cause back discomfort.

Shoulder and neck extensions need no equipment and can be done anywhere, making them a simple compliment to any workout regimen.

It is critical to remember that consistency is essential. This exercise, along with other focused back and core exercises, can considerably reduce back pain and improve general comfort and mobility in women over the age of 60. However, before beginning any fitness program, contact a healthcare practitioner to confirm it is safe and appropriate for your unique health needs.

Stretches for the Upper and Lower Back

Back pain is a common condition that can affect people of all ages, although it gets more common as we get older.

Women over the age of 60 are more prone to back discomfort due to factors such as decreasing bone density and muscle mass.

Fortunately, effective stretches that target both the upper and lower back can help ease back discomfort in this age range.

Stretches for the upper back: Squeeze your shoulder blades while standing or sitting up straight. Squeeze your shoulder blades together gently for 5–10 seconds. To improve upper back posture and alleviate stress, repeat 10 repetitions.

Neck Tilts: Tilt your head to the left and right for 15 seconds, holding each stretch. This aids in the release of tension in the neck and upper back.

Stretches for the Lower Back:
On your back lay with your knees bent. Hold one leg up to your chest for 15-20 seconds. Change legs. This stretch relieves lower back and sciatica discomfort.

Get on your hands and knees for the Cat-Cow Stretch. In a flowing motion, arch your back upward (cat) and then downward (cow). This increases lower back flexibility. Twist your spine:

Bend your knees and sit or lie down. Looking over your shoulder, gently shift your upper torso to one side.

Before repeating on the opposite side, hold for 15-20 seconds.

This stretch improves spine mobility, reducing lower and upper back pain.

Tilt of the Pelvis:

Lie down on your back with your legs bent.
With your lower back on the floor, tighten your abs.
Hold for a few seconds before releasing.
This exercise develops the muscles in the lower back.

The Child's Pose: Kneel on the floor and sit back on your heels, arms extended front. Hold this stretch for 20-30 seconds to allow your entire back to relax.

Always remember to stretch softly and regularly. These exercises can help you improve your posture, reduce muscle tension, and increase your general back flexibility, all of which contribute to a healthier, more comfortable back.

Before beginning any fitness regimen, consult with a healthcare physician, especially if you have any pre-existing medical concerns.

Exercises for Hip and Leg Mobility

Maintaining hip and leg mobility is critical for general health, especially as we become older.

These exercises can be especially beneficial for women in terms of controlling and avoiding back pain. Here are some helpful exercises for ladies to improve hip and leg mobility.

Stretch your hip flexors by squatting on one knee and gradually leaning forward until you feel a stretch in the front of your hip. Hold for 20–30 seconds before alternating sides.

This exercise relieves hip flexor tension, which can lead to back discomfort.

Swing one leg forth and backward while holding onto a sturdy surface. This action improves flexibility by increasing blood flow to the hip and leg muscles.

Sit in a chair with your back straight and perform seated leg lifts. Lift and hold one leg straight out in front of you for a few seconds. Lower it and do the same with the opposite leg.

This exercise develops the muscles in your legs, which helps to support your back.

Stretch your piriformis by sitting on the floor with your legs bent.

Cross one ankle over the opposing knee and press down softly on the lifted knee. You should feel a stretch in your buttocks, which will relieve strain on your lower back.

Standing Calf Raises: For support, stand behind a chair or counter. As you rise to your toes, drop your heels. This exercise helps to develop the calf muscles, which aids with balance and stability.

Tai Chi is an elegant Chinese technique that includes deep breathing and graceful motions. It's a great method to enhance your balance, flexibility, and leg strength, which all contribute to a healthy back.

Yoga: A variety of yoga positions help improve hip and leg mobility. Downward Dog, Warrior II, and Pigeon Pose all serve to stretch and develop these muscles.

Remember that consistency is essential. Include these exercises in your regular routine to progressively increase hip and leg mobility, which can aid in the relief and prevention of back pain.

Before beginning a new fitness regimen, always contact a healthcare practitioner, especially if you have any pre-existing health concerns.

Women can benefit from better mobility, less back discomfort, and an overall healthier lifestyle by devoting time to these activities.

Chapter 4 : Exercises to Strengthen Your Back

Maintaining excellent posture, lowering the risk of injury, and relieving back pain all need back strengthening.

This is especially crucial for women as they age, as the spine alters, causing pain and restricted mobility. We'll go over a variety of back-strengthening exercises for ladies over 60 in this article.

Cat-Cow Stretch: This yoga-inspired stretch improves spine flexibility.
Beggin on your hands and knees, arching your back upward (as if you were a cat) and then lowering it, elevating your head (as if you were a cow).

This mild motion can help relieve stiffness and improve spinal health.

Lie on your back with your knees bent and your feet flat on the floor for bridges. from your shoulders to your knees Create a straight line by lifting your hips.

This exercise focuses on the lower back and glutes, both of which are important for back stability.Lie on your stomach with your arms stretched front and your legs straight.

Lift your arms and legs off the ground at the same time, using your lower back muscles. This exercise is beneficial for strengthening the entire back.

Seated Row: Sit with your legs outstretched and your back erect, using resistance bands or weights.
 Squeeze your shoulder blades together and pull the resistance toward you. This exercise strengthens the upper back while also improving posture.

Wall Angels: Stand with your back to a wall and your arms at 90 degrees.

Slide your arms up and down the wall while keeping your head, shoulders, and lower back in touch.

This exercise improves shoulder mobility as well as upper back strength.

Planks: Core strength is essential for back support. The plank is a great option. With your weight on your forearms,Begin by doing a push-up.
Maintain a straight posture from head to heels, using your abdominal and lower back muscles.

Lie on your back with your legs bent. Tighten your abs and raise your pelvis, elevating your lower back slightly off the ground.

This exercise aids in the stabilization of the lower back and pelvis.

Before beginning any workout program, contact a healthcare practitioner or fitness expert, especially if you have pre-existing back pain or other issues.

These workouts may be tailored to your level of fitness, gradually increasing in intensity.

Regular exercise may considerably enhance your general well-being and lower your risk of back discomfort, ensuring that you remain active and healthy as you age.

Exercises to Strengthen Your Core

Core strength is essential for maintaining excellent posture, stability, and overall health, particularly as we age.

Back pain is a prevalent complaint among women, and including core-strengthening exercises into your regimen can help relieve pain and improve overall quality of life.

Planks: Begin in a simple plank posture, keeping your body straight from head to heels. Hold for as long as you can with your core muscles engaged. This workout strengthens your whole core and supports your spine.

Lie on your back with your knees bent and your feet flat on the floor for bridges. Squeeze your glutes and engage your core as you lift your hips off the ground. This exercise works the glutes and lower back.

Leg Raises: lift your legs straight up with your back on the floor

Slowly lower them without contacting the ground. This exercise works your lower abdominal muscles while also helping to support your lower back.

Sit on the floor with your knees bent and your feet flat for seated Russian twists.

Lean gently back, maintaining your back straight. While holding a weight or a household object, twist your torso from side to side. This exercise strengthens and stabilizes the oblique muscles.

Superman Pose: Lie down on your back with your arms and legs outstretched.

Lift your arms and legs off the ground at the same time, working your glutes and lower back. This workout helps to relieve back discomfort by strengthening the muscles along your spine.

Cat-Cow Stretch: Alternate between arching your back (like a cat) and rounding it (like a cow) on your hands and knees. This easy workout improves flexibility and reduces back stress.

It is critical to begin cautiously and progressively increasing the intensity of these workouts.

Listen to your body, and if you feel any discomfort or pain, stop and get medical attention.

Core strength is important for women, especially as they age, since it supports the back, improves posture, and can lower the risk of back discomfort dramatically.

Integrating these core-strengthening exercises into your workout program on a regular basis will help you maintain a healthy and pain-free back.

Strength Training for the Upper and Lower Bodies

Upper and lower body strength training is an important component of total health, especially for women who may be suffering from back discomfort.

While becoming older might provide its own set of obstacles, it's critical to focus on strength training to relieve and avoid back discomfort. Upper and lower body strengthening can improve posture, balance, and minimize the chance of injury.

Push-ups, dumbbell rows, and overhead presses are examples of upper body strength workouts.

These workouts not only develop strength but also help with posture, which can help with back discomfort.

Focusing on the upper back and shoulder muscles can help women, especially those over 60, offset the natural forward sag that occurs with aging.

This is especially good for individuals who sit for lengthy periods of time or have weak upper back muscles.

Squats, lunges, and leg presses are examples of lower body strength exercises. Lower-body strength not only supports the spine but also improves balance and movement.

Building strong leg muscles can help women with back pain maintain appropriate body mechanics and reduce the pressure on the lower back.

Individual requirements and restrictions must be considered while designing these activities. Injury can be avoided by beginning with modest weights and gradually increasing effort. A consultation with a healthcare practitioner or a fitness trainer who knows the unique requirements of women over the age of 60 suffering from back pain is a good first step.

Strength training, along with flexibility and aerobic routines, should be included in a well-rounded exercise plan for general health and pain management.

While becoming older might provide its own set of obstacles, committing to strength training can help women live more active, pain-free lives. Remember, it is never too late to begin, and the rewards are well worth the effort.

Posture and Balance Exercises

Maintaining proper posture and balance is critical for general health, particularly as we become older.

Back pain is a frequent problem for many people, and women, in particular, might suffer from it owing to a variety of circumstances.

Exercises that focus on posture and balance can considerably assist relieve and prevent back pain.

Posture Workouts: Shoulder Blade Squeeze: While sitting or standing, gently squeeze your shoulder blades together. It aids in the strengthening of the upper back muscles and the improvement of posture.

Hold for a few seconds and Tuck your chin inwards towards your chest

This exercise can help to offset the forward head position that is typically associated with back discomfort.

Standing with your back to a wall, gently lift your arms upwards, striving to contact the wall without arching your lower back. This practice encourages correct alignment.

Balance Workouts:

Single-Leg Stands: Stand for 30 seconds on one leg, then switch to the other. This easy exercise improves core strength and stability, lowering the chance of falling.

Heel-to-Toe Walk: Walk in a straight line with one foot in front of the other, heel to toe. This workout tests your balance and coordination.

Tai Chi: Think about taking a Tai Chi class. This traditional Chinese exercise promotes balance, flexibility, and relaxation by combining slow, flowing motions with deep breathing.

These are moderate workouts that may be adapted to various fitness levels.

Before beginning any new workout plan, ladies over the age of 60 should take it carefully and speak with a healthcare practitioner or fitness specialist.

Consistency is crucial, and these exercises can help improve posture, balance, and general back health over time, lowering the risk of back discomfort and improving quality of life.

Incorporating these posture and balance exercises into your regular routine will help you avoid back discomfort and live a healthy, active lifestyle. It's never too late to put your back health first and live a pain-free, active life.

Chapter 5: Cardiovascular Exercises with Minimal Impact

Maintaining an active lifestyle is critical for overall health, particularly as we get older. Regular exercise can be especially beneficial for women over 60 in terms of promoting cardiovascular health and weight management.

However, back pain can make it difficult to choose appropriate exercises. Fortunately, there are a variety of cardiovascular exercises that provide a good workout while having little impact on the back.

Swimming is an excellent option for women suffering from back pain. The buoyancy of the water supports your body, reducing back strain. Water aerobics or leisurely laps can help you improve your cardiovascular fitness without the jarring impact of high-impact exercises.

Cycling on a stationary bike is yet another low-impact option.

It is easy on the spine and allows you to control the intensity of your workout. While benefiting from an effective cardiovascular exercise, adjust the resistance to match your fitness level.

Walking is a simple but extremely effective cardiovascular exercise. Wear comfortable, supportive shoes, and choose smooth, even surfaces.

A brisk walk can raise your heart rate and help you manage your weight while lowering your risk of back pain exacerbations.

Elliptical Trainer: The elliptical trainer is a low-impact, full-body workout machine. It's gentle on the joints and ideal for women who want to improve their cardiovascular health without putting too much strain on their backs.

Rowing machines provide a unique cardiovascular workout that engages multiple muscle groups.

The fluid, rhythmic motion reduces stress on the spine, making it an excellent choice for those suffering from back pain.

Tai Chi is a low-impact exercise that combines slow movements with deep breathing. It has the potential to improve cardiovascular fitness, flexibility, and balance while being gentle on the back.

It is critical to consult with a healthcare professional before beginning any exercise routine, especially if you have existing back pain or other health concerns. They can offer advice and ensure that the exercises you choose are safe and appropriate for your specific needs.

Incorporating these low-impact cardiovascular exercises into your fitness routine can help you maintain cardiovascular health, manage your weight, and lower your risk of back pain aggravation.

Staying active is an important part of aging well, and these exercises can help you do just that.

Advantages of Exercise for the Heart

Exercise is essential for maintaining cardiovascular health in women of all ages. However, as women age, they are more prone to a variety of health problems, including back pain.

Regular exercise has numerous benefits for the heart, and it also plays an important role in managing and preventing back pain.

Exercise, first and foremost, strengthens the heart muscle.

Cardiovascular exercises, such as brisk walking, jogging, or swimming, improve the efficiency with which the heart pumps blood.

A strong heart can pump more blood with each beat, requiring less effort to deliver oxygen and nutrients to the body's tissues.

This decreased workload on the heart reduces the risk of heart disease.

Exercise also improves blood circulation throughout the body, including the back muscles and structures.

Improved circulation aids in the delivery of essential nutrients to the spine and its surrounding tissues, which can aid in the prevention or relief of back pain.

Furthermore, regular physical activity helps with weight management, which is important for both heart health and reducing back pain.

Maintaining a healthy weight reduces the strain on the spine and lowers the risk of conditions such as osteoarthritis and herniated discs, both of which commonly cause back pain.

Exercise has also been shown to reduce stress and anxiety, both of which can contribute to heart problems and back pain.

Physical activity releases endorphins, which are natural mood elevators, resulting in an improved overall sense of well-being.

Exercise has numerous heart-health benefits, including the prevention and management of back pain in women.

It helps to maintain a healthy heart and a pain-free back by strengthening the heart, improving circulation, assisting with weight management, and reducing stress.

As a result, women of all ages should incorporate regular exercise into their routines to reap these benefits and live a healthier, more active life.

Nordic Walking and lWalking

Back pain is a common problem that affects people of all ages, but it can be especially difficult for women as they age. Low-impact exercises such as Nordic walking and regular walking, on the other hand, can be excellent choices for back pain management.

These activities not only give you a gentle cardiovascular workout, but they also help to strengthen the muscles that support your spine.

Nordic Walking, also known as pole walking, is a full-body exercise that involves walking while holding specially designed walking poles.

This type of exercise works the upper body, which helps to improve posture and balance. Nordic Walking is beneficial to women over the age of 60 because it relieves pressure on the lower back while promoting better spinal alignment.

Walking, on the other hand, is a simple and easy way to stay active.

A brisk walk can offer many of the same benefits as Nordic Walking, such as improved circulation and muscle tone.

The key is to walk with good posture, which helps to relieve strain on the lower back.

Both types of walking can be tailored to an individual's fitness level and degree of back pain.

Starting slowly and gradually increasing the intensity and duration of these exercises is critical. Proper footwear and clothing are also required for a safe and enjoyable experience.
It is best to consult with a healthcare professional or a fitness instructor who

specializes in back pain exercise. They can provide tailored guidance and exercises based on your specific needs and limitations.

Nordic walking and regular walking are great low-impact exercises for women who suffer from back pain.

They can boost overall fitness, strengthen core muscles, and relieve back pain, all of which contribute to a higher quality of life.

Incorporating these activities into your daily routine can help you achieve a healthier, pain-free back.

Hydrotherapy and Aquatic Exercises

Back pain is a common ailment that can have a significant impact on a person's quality of life, particularly as they get older.

Women, in particular, are more prone to back pain, and those over 60 frequently face additional challenges.

Hydrotherapy and aquatic exercises have emerged as effective treatments for back pain in this population. This gentle and supportive form of exercise has a number of advantages for women who are suffering from back pain.

The buoyancy of water is critical in hydrotherapy and aquatic exercises.

It lessens the impact on joints, making it an excellent choice for older people, including women over 60, who may suffer from age-related joint issues.

Water's buoyancy supports the body, relieving pressure on the spine and encouraging flexibility and movement without causing additional strain.

Furthermore, the natural resistance of water challenges muscles, resulting in increased strength and endurance.

Warm water pool hydrotherapy exercises are especially effective for back pain. The warm water relaxes muscles and increases blood circulation, promoting healing and pain relief.

Walking, leg lifts, and gentle stretches are all simple movements that can be tailored to an individual's fitness level and specific needs.
These exercises help to stabilize the core, which is important for managing back pain.

Aquatic exercises, which range from swimming to water aerobics, provide a comprehensive approach to back pain relief. Swimming, in particular, engages multiple muscle groups while improving cardiovascular fitness and being gentle on the back.

Water aerobics classes can offer a structured and social setting for women to engage in low-impact exercises that focus on core strength and overall well-being.

Women over the age of 60 who are suffering from back pain can benefit from hydrotherapy and aquatic exercises.

These activities can help you improve your flexibility, strength, and circulation while lowering your risk of injury.

They provide an enjoyable and safe way for older people to stay active and manage their back pain, ultimately improving their overall quality of life.

Chapter 6: Relieving Back Pain with Yoga and Tai Chi

Back pain becomes a common and often debilitating issue as we age, particularly for women.
Gentle exercises such as yoga and tai chi, on the other hand, can provide significant relief and improve overall well-being.

These practices provide a comprehensive approach to back pain relief, addressing both physical discomfort and mental stress.

Yoga, an ancient practice, emphasizes flexibility, strength, and relaxation.

It includes a variety of poses and stretches that can be tailored to the needs of individuals, including women over the age of 60.

Many of these postures, including cat-cow, Child's Pose, and Bridge, gently lengthen the spine, increase flexibility, and reduce back muscle tension.

Furthermore, the deep breathing and meditation aspects of Yoga aid in the management of stress, which can aggravate back pain.

Another ancient practice, Tai Chi, emphasizes slow, flowing movements that improve balance and stability. Controlled, low-impact motions are ideal for seniors and can help relieve back pain.

Tai Chi strengthens the core muscles and improves posture, reducing spinal strain. Its meditative aspect also aids in stress reduction and relaxation, which can be beneficial in the management of chronic pain.

A combination of Yoga and Tai Chi can be especially effective in addressing the unique challenges that women over 60 face.

These exercises are easy on the joints, promote flexibility, and gradually build strength without putting the body under undue strain. Consistency is essential, and regular practice can result in long-term relief.

It is critical to consult with a healthcare professional before beginning any exercise regimen to ensure that these activities are safe and appropriate for your specific condition.

Furthermore, seeking guidance from certified instructors with experience working with seniors can assist in tailoring the exercises to individual needs and limitations.

Yoga and Tai Chi are effective methods for relieving back pain in women over the age of 60.

These practices take a holistic approach to pain management, addressing not only the physical but also the mental and emotional aspects.

Many women can experience significant relief and live a more active and pain-free life by incorporating these gentle exercises into their daily routine.

An Overview of Tai Chi and Yoga

Back pain becomes a common and often debilitating issue as we age, particularly for women.

Gentle exercises such as yoga and tai chi, on the other hand, can provide significant relief and improve overall well-being.

These practices provide a comprehensive approach to back pain relief, addressing both physical discomfort and mental stress.

Yoga, an ancient practice, emphasizes flexibility, strength, and relaxation.

It includes a variety of poses and stretches that can be tailored to the needs of individuals, including women over the age of 60.

Many of these postures, including cat-cow, Child's Pose, and Bridge, gently lengthen the spine, increase flexibility, and reduce back muscle tension. Furthermore, the deep breathing and meditation aspects of Yoga aid in the management of stress, which can aggravate back pain.

Another ancient practice, Tai Chi, emphasizes slow, flowing movements that improve balance and stability.

Controlled, low-impact motions are ideal for seniors and can help relieve back pain. Tai Chi strengthens the core muscles and improves posture, reducing spinal strain.

Its meditative aspect also aids in stress reduction and relaxation, which can be beneficial in the management of chronic pain.
A combination of Yoga and Tai Chi can be especially effective in addressing the unique challenges that women over 60 face. These exercises are easy on the joints, promote flexibility, and gradually build strength

without putting the body under undue strain. Consistency is essential, and regular practice can result in long-term relief.

It is critical to consult with a healthcare professional before beginning any exercise regimen to ensure that these activities are safe and appropriate for your specific condition.

Furthermore, seeking guidance from certified instructors with experience working with seniors can assist in tailoring the exercises to individual needs and limitations.

Yoga and Tai Chi are effective methods for relieving back pain in women over the age of 60.

These practices take a holistic approach to pain management, addressing not only the physical but also the mental and emotional aspects.

Many women can experience significant relief and live a more active and pain-free life by incorporating these gentle exercises into their daily routine.

Back Health Pose and Movement Techniques

Maintaining a healthy back is important at any age, but it becomes even more important as we get older.

Back pain affects many people, particularly women, and certain exercises and movement techniques can significantly improve back health.

In this section, we'll look at some back pain exercise techniques for women that are both beneficial and age-appropriate.

Gentle stretching exercises are ideal for women over the age of 60. These stretches improve flexibility and reduce muscle tension, which can help relieve back pain. Incorporate movements like the cat-cow stretch, in which you slowly arch and round your back. This improves spinal mobility and relieves stress.

Core Strengthening: A strong core provides spinal support. Exercises that target the abdominal muscles, such as pelvic tilts and seated leg lifts, should be done. These can assist in stabilizing your back and lowering your risk of injury.

Low-Impact Cardio: Walking or swimming are low-impact aerobic exercises that can improve overall fitness without putting too much strain on the back. This improves circulation and reduces inflammation.

Yoga and Pilates: Both yoga and Pilates offer core strength, balance, and flexibility exercises. These exercises are ideal for women who want to improve their back health and posture.

Proper Posture Awareness: It is critical to develop an awareness of your posture. Sit and stand with your spine neutral and aligned. To avoid unnecessary strain on your back, avoid slouching or prolonged periods of poor posture.

Body Mechanics: Learn to lift objects properly by bending at the hips and knees rather than at the waist. This reduces the likelihood of back injuries during everyday activities.

Consult a Professional: Before beginning any exercise regimen, it is critical to consult a healthcare professional or a physical therapist, especially if you have existing back pain or medical conditions.

When it comes to back health, remember that consistency is everything.

These exercises and movement techniques should be done on a regular basis to reap long-term benefits. Women can enjoy better back health, less pain, and a higher quality of life as they age if they take the right approach.

Relaxation Breathing Methods

Relaxation breathing techniques are an important tool for managing back pain, especially for women.

Our bodies change as we age, and for women, this often includes musculoskeletal issues such as back pain.

Fortunately, there are effective relaxation breathing techniques that can relieve pain and improve overall well-being.

Deep diaphragmatic breathing is one of the most commonly recommended relaxation breathing methods for back pain..

This technique entails taking slow, deep breaths while focusing on diaphragm expansion rather than shallow chest breathing.

You are engaging the diaphragm and helping to relax the muscles surrounding the spine, reducing tension and pain. Experiment with this method by inhaling for four counts, holding for four counts, and exhaling for four counts, gradually increasing the duration as your comfort level improves.

Progressive muscle relaxation is another useful breathing technique that combines deep breathing with muscle relaxation.

Begin by taking a deep breath, then as you exhale, consciously release tension in specific muscle groups, working your way up from your toes to your neck and shoulders.

This technique encourages muscle relaxation and reduces the strain that frequently aggravates back pain.

Mindfulness meditation is another effective method for dealing with back pain. You can reduce stress, which is known to contribute to pain perception, by focusing your attention on your breath and the present moment. Regular mindfulness meditation practice can also help your body's natural ability to heal and regenerate.

Relaxation breathing techniques provide a comprehensive approach to treating female back pain.

These techniques can help to relieve discomfort, improve posture, and reduce the emotional burden that chronic pain often brings.

Women can empower themselves to better manage and potentially alleviate their back pain by incorporating these methods into their daily routine, improving their quality of life as they age.

Chapter 7: Establishing a Long-Term Workout Schedule

Creating a Long-Term Workout Schedule for Women's Back Pain Relief

Back discomfort is a frequent problem for women of all ages, but it may be especially difficult for women over 60.

Our bodies change as we age, and keeping a healthy back becomes even more important.

Fortunately, with the correct workout plan, it is possible to relieve back pain while also maintaining a strong, flexible spine.

It is critical to focus on activities that enhance flexibility, strength, and general well-being while developing a long-term fitness routine for back pain alleviation.

Here's a detailed guide on developing an effective training routine:

Speak with a healthcare professional: Before beginning any fitness program, speak with your healthcare practitioner to confirm that the workouts you choose are safe for your specific health concerns.

Stretching exercises can help increase flexibility and minimize the chance of muscular strains. Incorporate shoulder rolls, neck stretches, and mild twists into your workout program.

Strengthen your core: A strong core gives back support. In order to target the muscles that support your spine, use movements such as planks, bridges, and leg lifts.

Low-impact cardio exercises such as walking, swimming, or stationary cycling can improve circulation and reduce stiffness without putting strain on your back.

Mindful posture: Pay attention to your posture as you go about your everyday tasks. Back discomfort may be avoided by keeping a straight back and good alignment.

Gradual progression means that you should begin slowly and progressively increase the intensity and duration of your workouts. Avoid overexertion by listening to your body.

Consistency is essential: Make a training routine and aim for at least 150 minutes of moderate-intensity activity every week.

Maintain a balanced diet and stay hydrated: Proper nutrition and hydration are vital for general health and can help your workout schedule.

Seek expert advice: Consider working with a licensed fitness trainer or physical therapist who can customize a training plan for you and give coaching to guarantee appropriate form.

You may successfully treat back pain and live a more active and pain-free life by following these instructions and making a long-term commitment to your training plan.

Making Reasonable Objectives

Setting acceptable goals for back pain exercises is critical, especially for ladies over the age of 60.

Prioritizing the individual's well-being and health is critical, with objectives tailored to their personal requirements and constraints. Here are some crucial aspects for setting appropriate goals for back pain exercise:

Assess Current Condition: Before establishing any goals, it is critical to assess the individual's current condition of health and back discomfort. Existing medical ailments or injuries It is critical to understand where you are beginning from.

Consult a Healthcare expert: It is best to get advice from a healthcare expert or physical therapist. They can make tailored advice and assist in establishing safe and effective objectives.

Pain Management: The primary goal should be pain alleviation and management. Reduced back pain intensity and frequency should take precedence over more ambitious fitness objectives.

Flexibility and Mobility: It is critical to work on enhancing flexibility and mobility. Stretching exercises can aid in the reduction of stiffness and the expansion of the range of motion in the back and surrounding muscles.

Strength and Posture: It is critical to strengthen the core and back muscles for stability and support. However, goals in this area should be set with discretion in order to avoid overexertion.

Gradual Progression: Goals should be progressive and attainable. It is critical to begin at a low intensity and progressively raise as the individual grows more familiar with the exercises.

Consistency is essential for success. Setting goals for a consistent exercise regimen, even if only a few times per week, may considerably improve general back health.

Monitor Progress: Monitor progress on a regular basis and alter objectives as appropriate. The individual's condition may change over time, and the workout routine must be adjusted accordingly.

Enjoyment and Mental Well-being: Do not underestimate the value of enjoyment and mental well-being. Setting goals connected to having fun while exercising can help with program adherence.

Integrating Back Pain Exercises into Daily living: The ultimate objective should be to include back pain exercises into daily living. The goals of incorporating exercise into one's lifestyle are both sensible and helpful.

Setting realistic goals for back pain exercises for women over 60 should be based on their individual requirements, restrictions, and ambitions.

It is critical to prioritize pain management, flexibility, and progressive improvement in order to improve their overall well-being and quality of life.

Consultation with healthcare specialists and regularity in their workout program might help them achieve their fitness objectives even more effectively.

Creating a Weekly Workout Schedule

Back discomfort is a frequent complaint among women, and it can worsen as we age.

A regular exercise program, particularly for women over the age of 60, can assist ease pain and boost general health.

Consider the following principles when creating an effective weekly training routine to alleviate back discomfort.

1. Consult a healthcare professional: Before starting any new workout regimen, talk to your doctor, especially if you have back problems. They can give individualized advice and propose appropriate workouts.

2. Concentrate on flexibility and strength: Include activities that improve flexibility and strengthen the muscles that support your back. Stretching, light yoga, or resistance training may be included.

3. *Prioritize posture:* Pay attention to your posture when exercising and going about your regular activities. Proper posture may drastically minimize back discomfort. Make sure your training program incorporates posture and alignment exercises.

4. *Cardiovascular activity:* Walk, swim, or cycle for low-impact cardiovascular exercise. Cardiovascular activity improves general health and aids in the maintenance of a healthy weight, which can reduce the strain on your back.

5. *Gradual progression:* Begin slowly and progressively raise your workout intensity. Excessive exercise can aggravate back discomfort, so be aware of your body's limits.

6. *Consistency:* Aim for 150 minutes of moderate-intensity activity each week, but divide it up into manageable sessions. The key to receiving the rewards is consistency.

7. *Rest and recovery:* Give your body time to rest and heal in between sessions. Adequate rest is critical for healing and injury prevention.

8. *range:* To avoid boredom and to stimulate different muscle areas, use a range of activities. In order to make your workouts more appealing, incorporate things that you like.

9. *Pay attention to your body:* If a workout causes pain or discomfort, stop immediately and see your doctor. Replace or modify the activity to make it more pleasant.

10. *Keep track of your progress:* Keep track of your workouts and how your back feels. This will allow you to track your progress and make any required changes to your program.

Creating a weekly training routine for women over 60 to relieve back pain involves careful preparation and consideration to individual needs.

Maintaining a healthy, pain-free back requires consistency, appropriate form, and regular check-ins with your healthcare professional.

Maintaining Drive and Changing With Time

Physical health and well-being are essential at any age. Women, particularly those over the age of 60, frequently confront specific obstacles in maintaining their general health, particularly when it comes to treating back pain.

Back discomfort is a typical complaint among older folks, but it should not prevent them from being active and mobile.

Consistency and adaptation are the keys to properly treating back pain and maintaining motivation.

First and foremost, workout consistency is critical.

Regular exercise can help to strengthen the muscles that support the spine and relieve back discomfort. Women over the age of 60 should engage in a variety of aerobic, strength training, and flexibility exercises.

This continuous program can result in enhanced endurance, less discomfort, and better overall health.

However, it's critical to remember that as we get older, our bodies change, and so do our activity requirements.

What worked in our youth may not be appropriate anymore. The second critical component of controlling back pain is adaptability.

Women over the age of 60 should pay attention to their bodies and be open to change their workout regimens as required.

Low-impact workouts like swimming and mild yoga can be gentler on aging joints and muscles, lowering the chance of injury.

It is also critical to get advice from healthcare specialists and competent trainers.

They may create customized workout routines based on an individual's demands and limits, ensuring that the exercises are both safe and effective.

Maintaining motivation and adjusting to changing body demands are critical components in controlling back pain via exercise for women without allowing age to become a limiting factor.

Regular, adapted exercise programs can help women over the age of 60 stay active, relieve back discomfort, and live a healthier, more happy life.

These ladies may age gracefully while taking care of their physical well-being by establishing a balance between constancy and adaptability.

CONCLUSION

Finally, back pain exercises are extremely beneficial for ladies who want to keep a healthy and active lifestyle as they age. These exercises provide a holistic approach to reducing pain and improving general well-being.

Developing strong back muscles and flexibility, regardless of age, is critical for preventing and alleviating back discomfort. These workouts are especially important for ladies over the age of 60.

The aging process frequently causes changes in bone density and muscle mass, making the back more prone to pain.

A personalized workout plan that focuses on back strengthening, posture improvement, and flexibility can successfully offset these age-related difficulties. Furthermore, frequent physical exercise improves bone health and circulation, aiding in the prevention of chronic pain and promoting a healthy lifestyle.

It is critical to emphasize that before beginning any fitness program, especially for people of this age, you should check with a healthcare expert.

They may make tailored recommendations and verify that the workouts are safe and fit for the individual's demands and circumstances.

Overall, back pain exercises enable women to age gracefully, remain independent, and completely enjoy life.

Women may take charge of their back health and enjoy the numerous advantages of an active, pain-free lifestyle by adopting these exercises into their everyday lives.

THANK YOU PAGE

Thank you for choosing "Back Pain Exercises for Women Over 60." Your help is much appreciated! We respect your comments and would appreciate it if you could submit a review. Your feedback will assist us in improving and creating even better material for our upcoming book.

Cheers to a Healthy you!!!

Printed in Great Britain
by Amazon

43537963R00066